The Glitter Heart
A Story of Resilience

Story by Valerie E. Sifuentes
Art by Yvette Koebke

The Glitter Heart
A story of resilience

Copyright © 2020, Independently Published via KDP

ISBN: 9798668238675

Audrey's Aura
www.audreysaura.com

Yvette Koebke Art
https://www.facebook.com/yvettekoebkeart/

All Rights Reserved. No part of this text may be reproduced, stored in a retrieval system, or transmitted by any means, electronic, mechanical, photocopying, desktop publishing, recording, or otherwise, without permission from the publisher. No patent liability is assumed with respect to the use of the information contained herein. While every precaution has been taken in the preparation of this book, the publisher and author assume no responsibility for errors or omissions. Neither is any liability assumed for damages resulting from the use of the information contained

This book is dedicated to the caring staff at
Children's Hospital Los Angeles
A special thank you to
Dr. Kristopher Kallin and
Dr. Joseph Mares of
Kaiser Permenante
for taking care of Audrey's
glitter heart with
such grace and compassion.

There is a girl named Audrey.
When she was 4 years old,
she loved to sing, she loved to dance,
with a glitter heart of gold.

She shimmered in the sun.
She sparkled in the night.
She loved to tell spooky stories with
a smile big and bright.

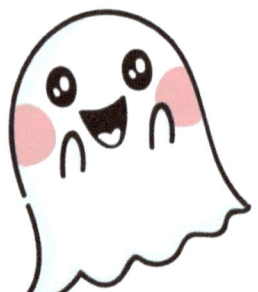

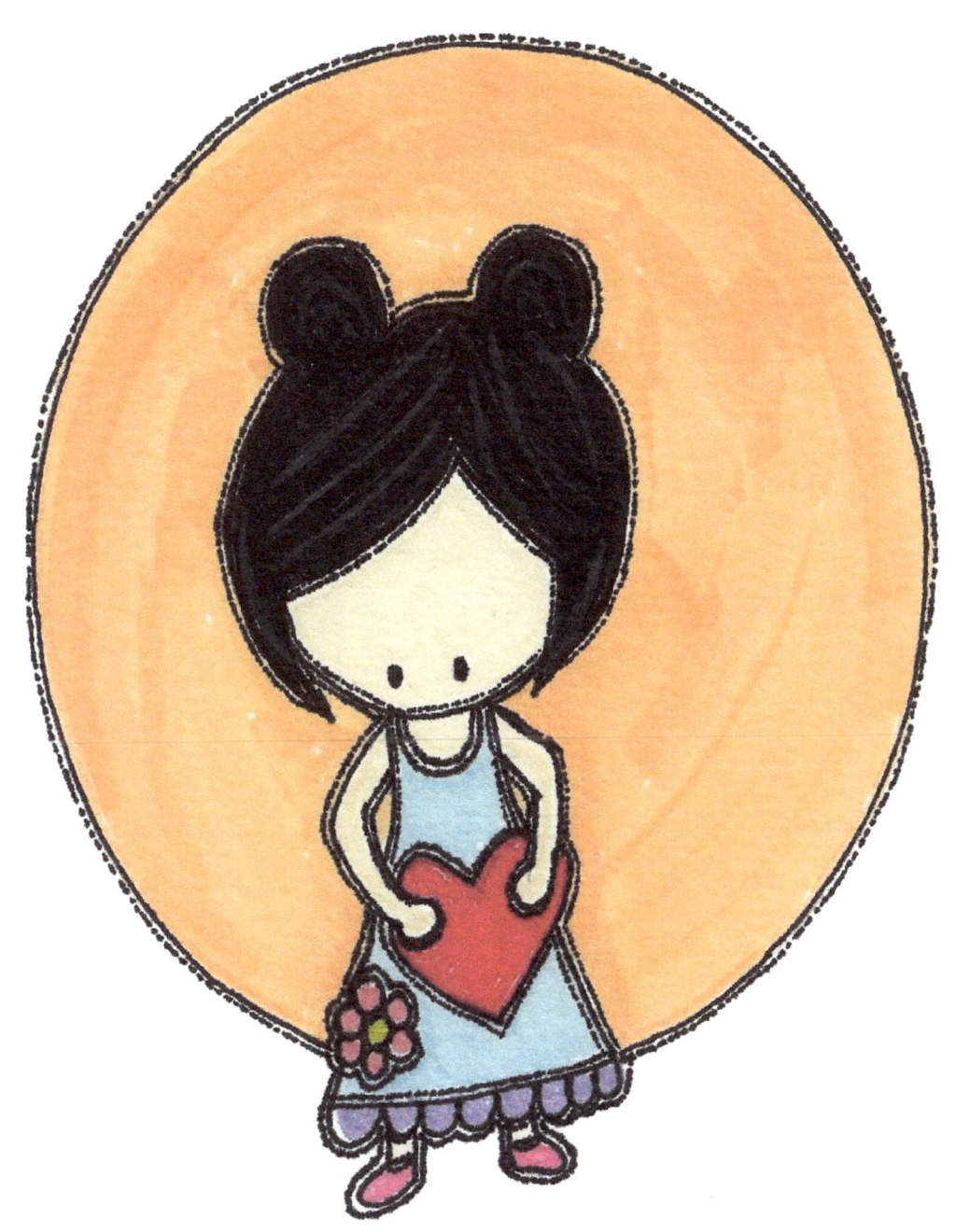

To look at her you would think,
She was a healthy child.
So funny and so energetic,
Always running wild.

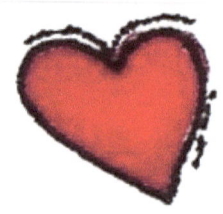

But what others did not know,
Is that when this glitter girl was born,
Her heart...it made a special sound,
like a soft trumpet horn.

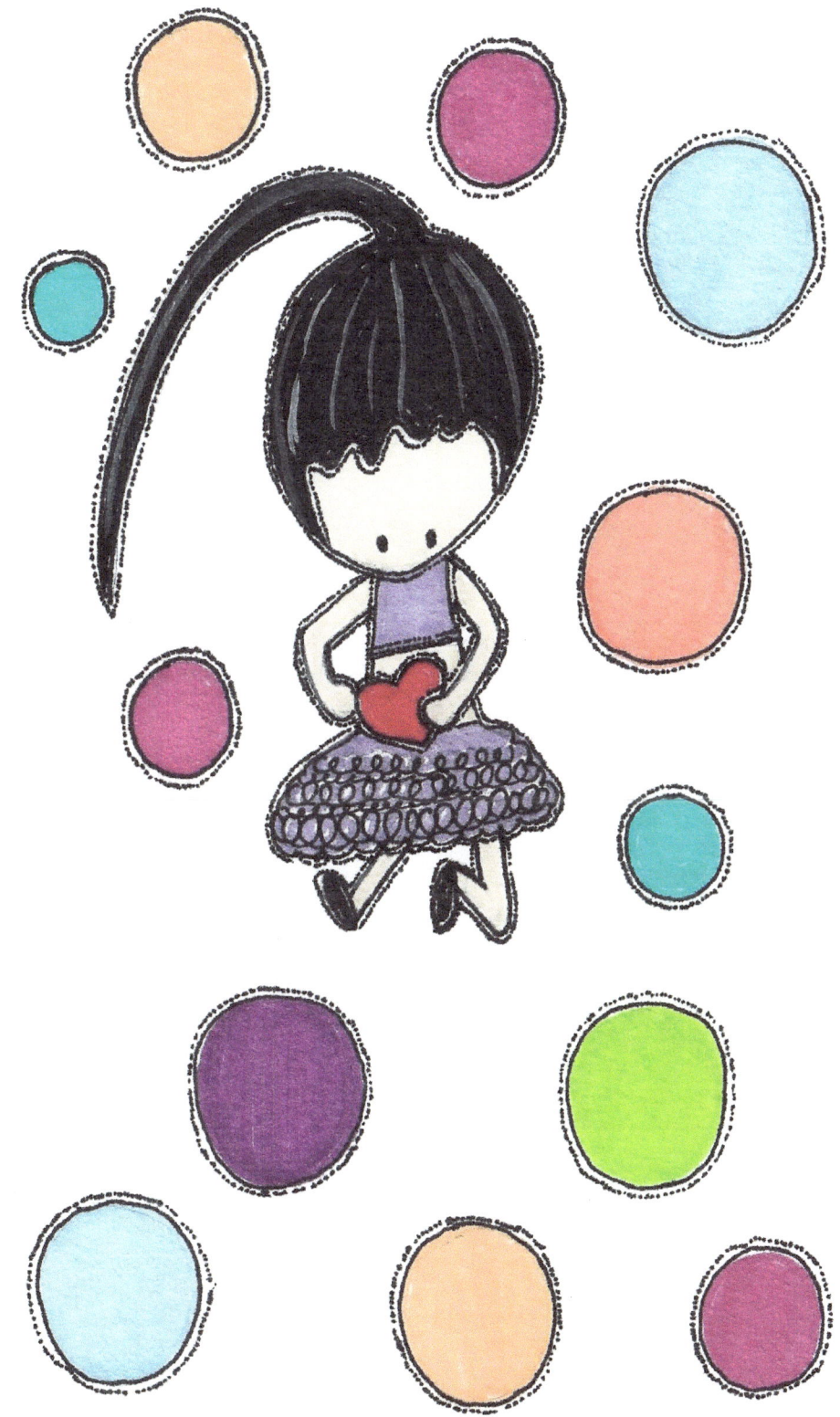

They said not to worry, do not fret.

She's a strong and mighty girl,

with a spirit oh so colorful

it creates a glitter whirl.

When Audrey soon grew older,

They looked deep down in her heart.

They found a tiny hole inside it

that created quite a spark!

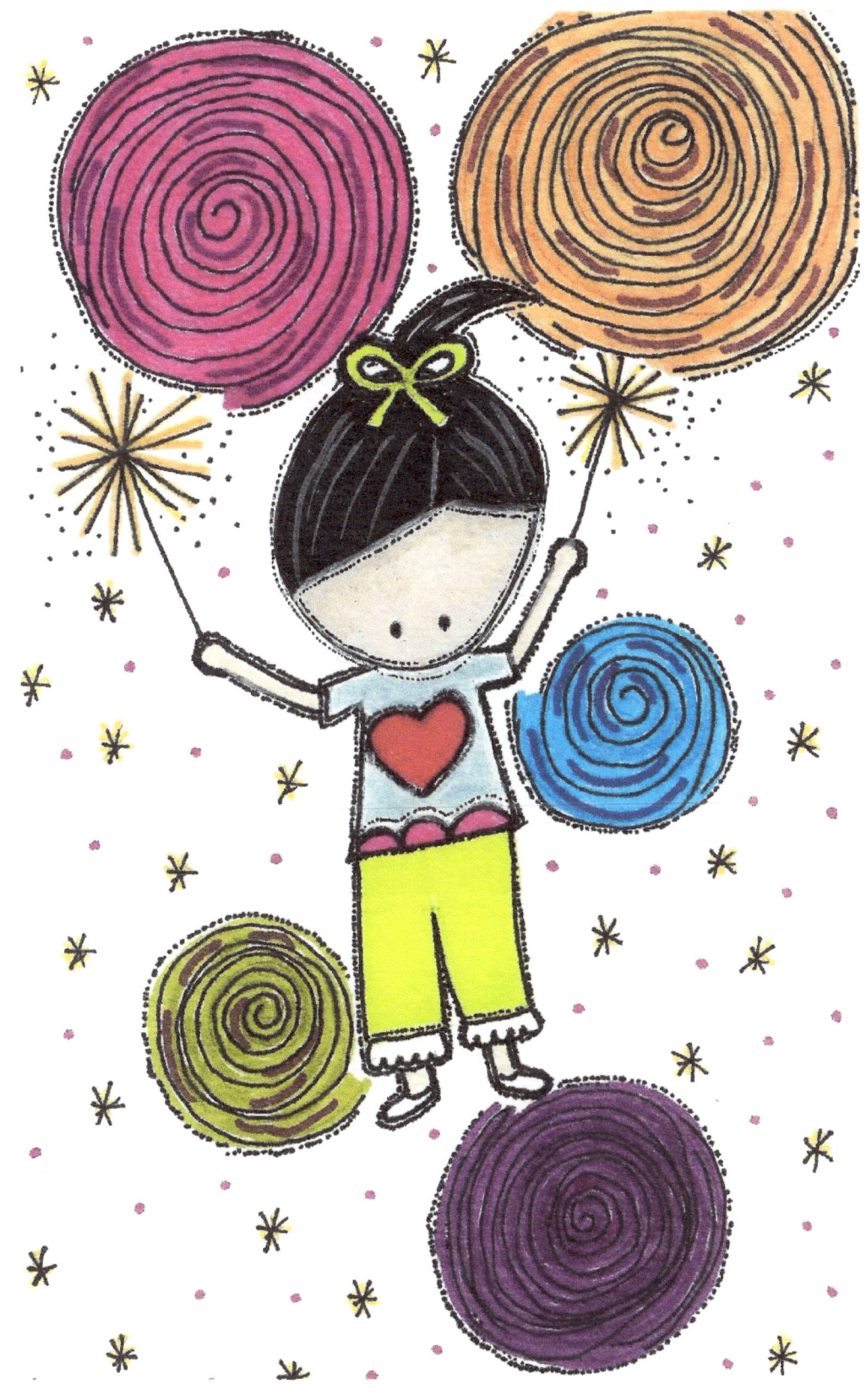

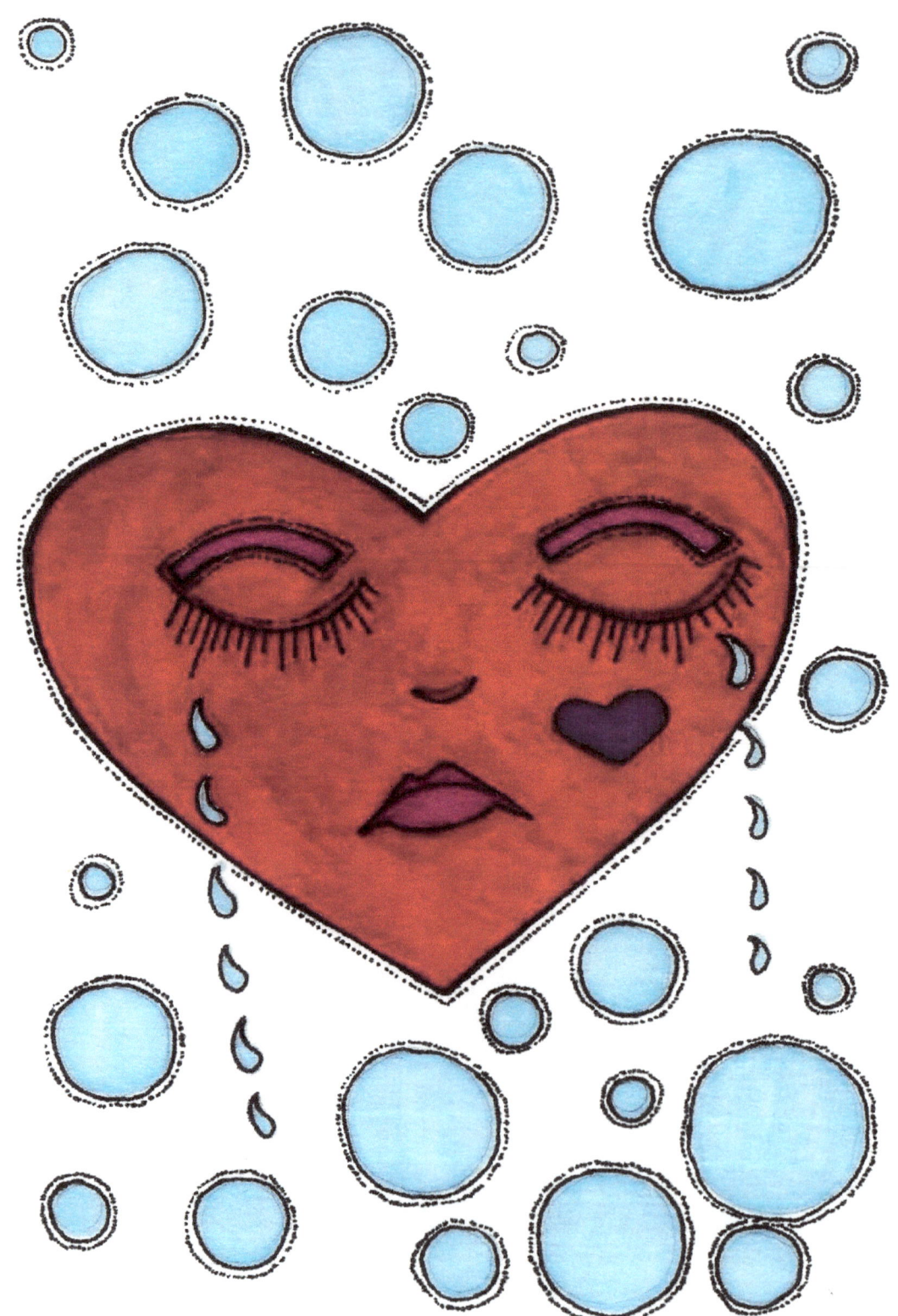

She never showed a sign of sickness
Or feeling bad at all.
So, this created quite the wonder
When doctors came to call.

But you see, the glitter from her heart
Leaked from one side to the next,
The doctors went to work so fast
and did a bunch of tests!

Her Mommy and her Daddy said.
Don't you worry now my sweet,
They are going fix your glitter,
So that heart won't skip a beat.

When the morning came
and it was time to go in,
She was Spooky, Scared and Sad
for the surgery to begin.

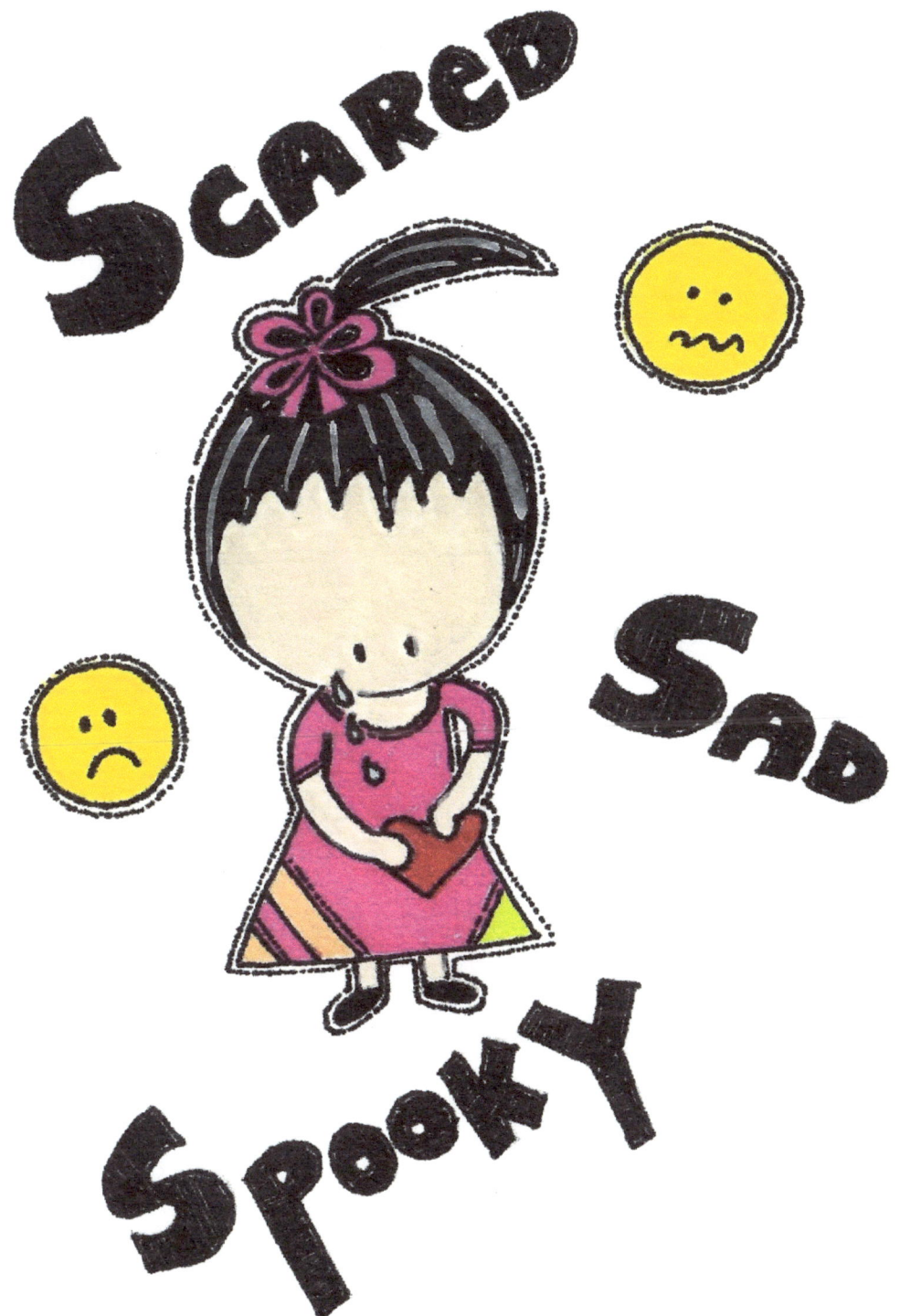

Take a deep breath...
Her Mommy said.
It will soon be over
And you'll be comfy in bed!

The time was soon here,
and she fell asleep quick.
She felt nothing at all,
As her heartbeat was fixed.

Her Mommy, Daddy and family
All prayed, prayed and prayed.
She woke up at last!
Her glitter was saved!!

Her heart stopped leaking!
Everyone breathed at last!
Her love beats on!
The worst had passed.

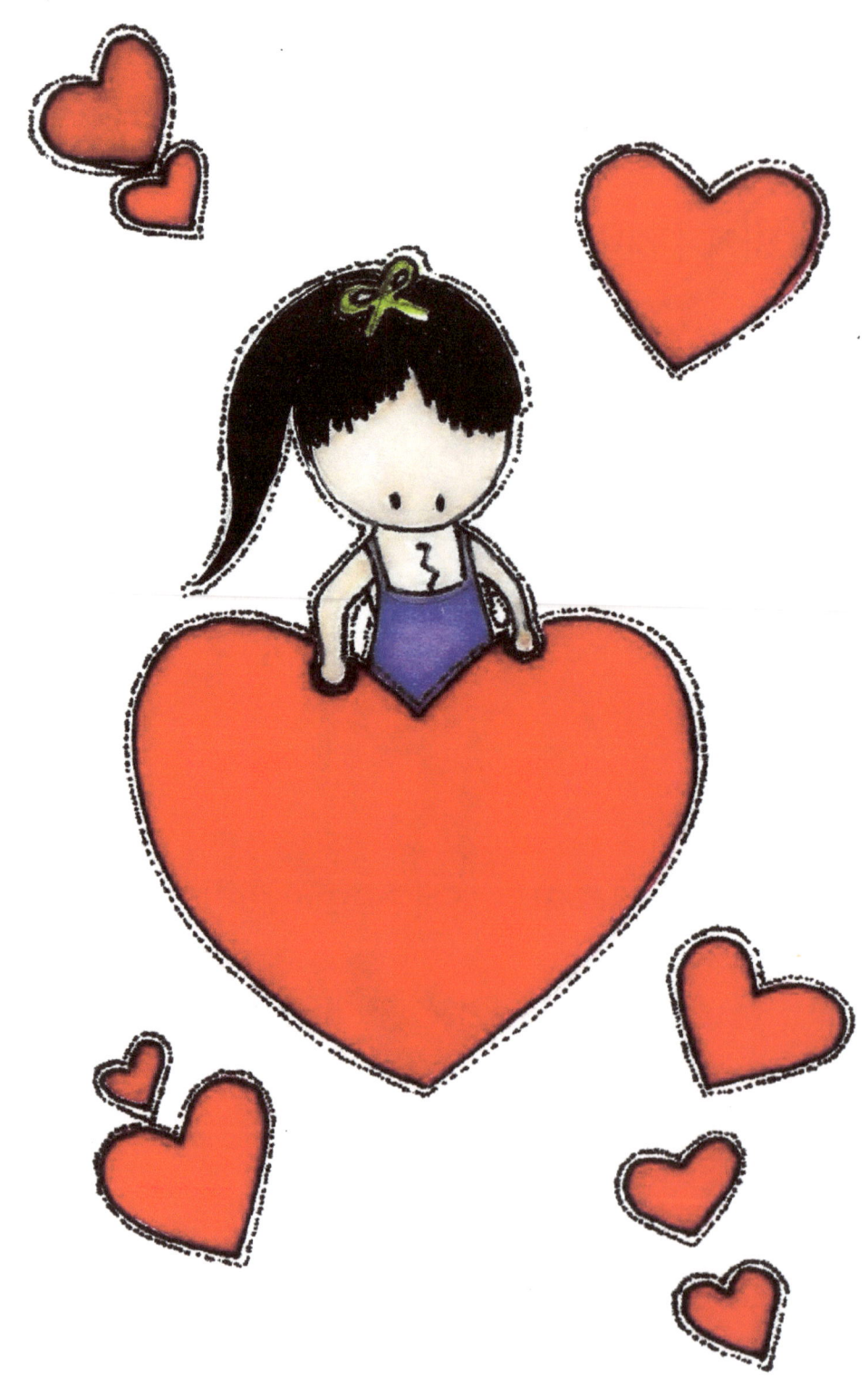

Yes, it's all over.
The time is gone.
But through it all,
the memory lives on.

Now a special scar
lives upon her chest,
it marks her special journey
a symbol of her healing quest.

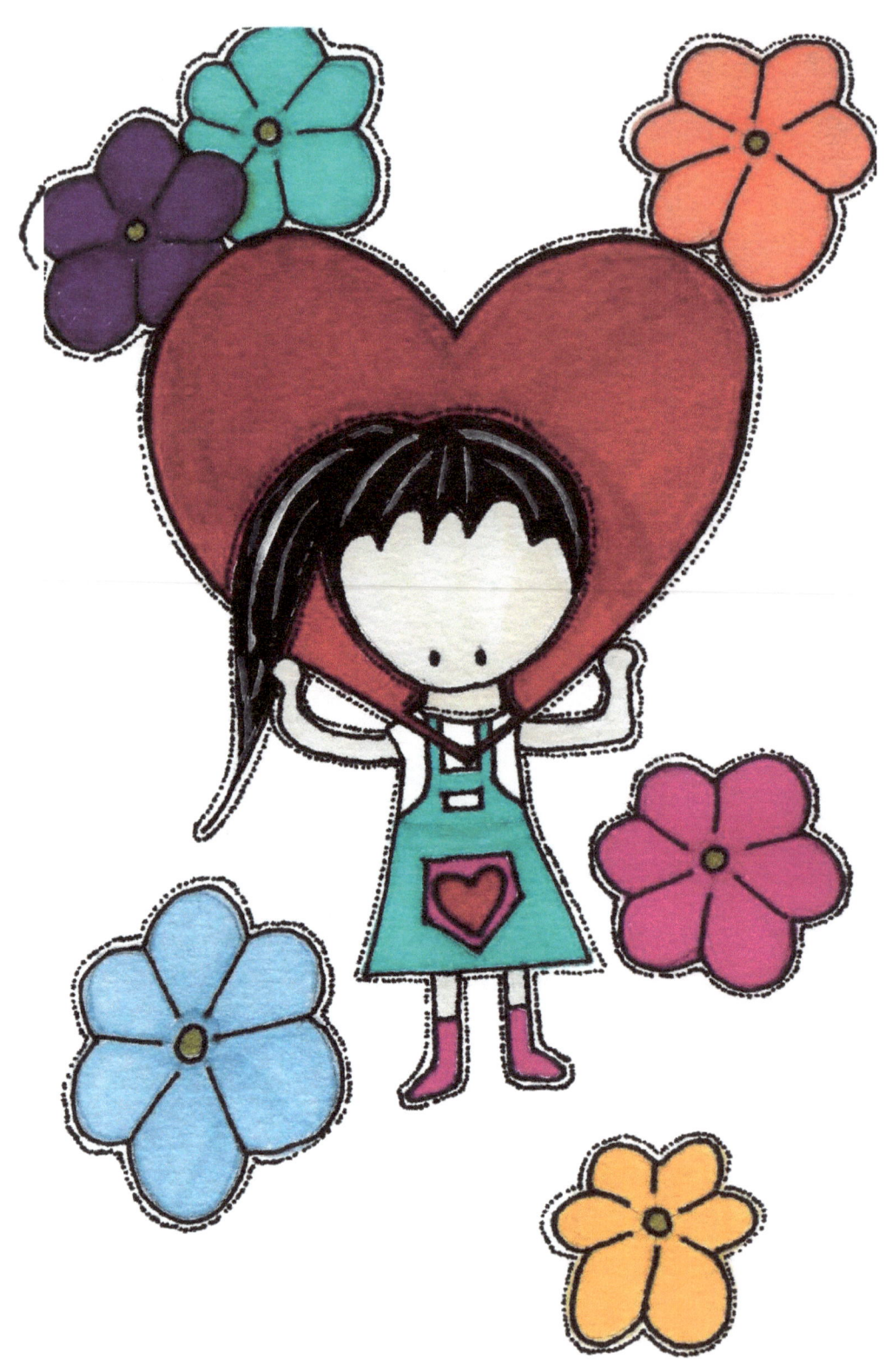

Audrey is as strong and brave
As anyone can be.

No matter if she's dancing.
Or slaying dragons in the sea.

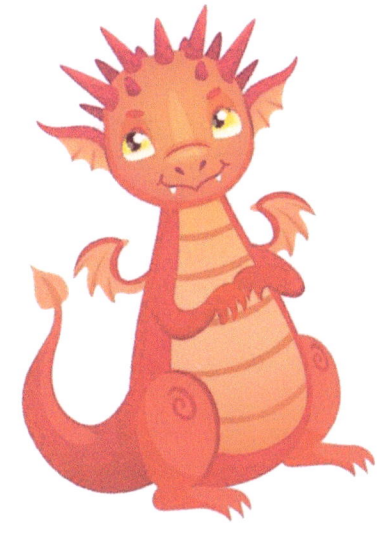
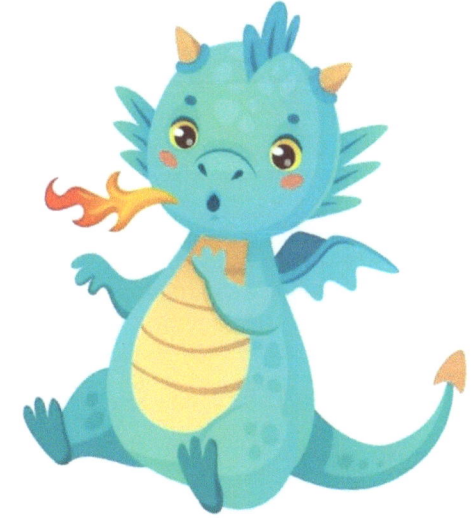

Because on a that magical
day her life was saved.
Soon she did turn five.

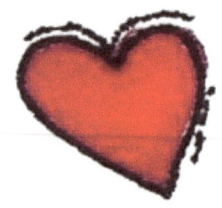

Happy, healthy, and full of life,
with a glitter heart
that thrives!

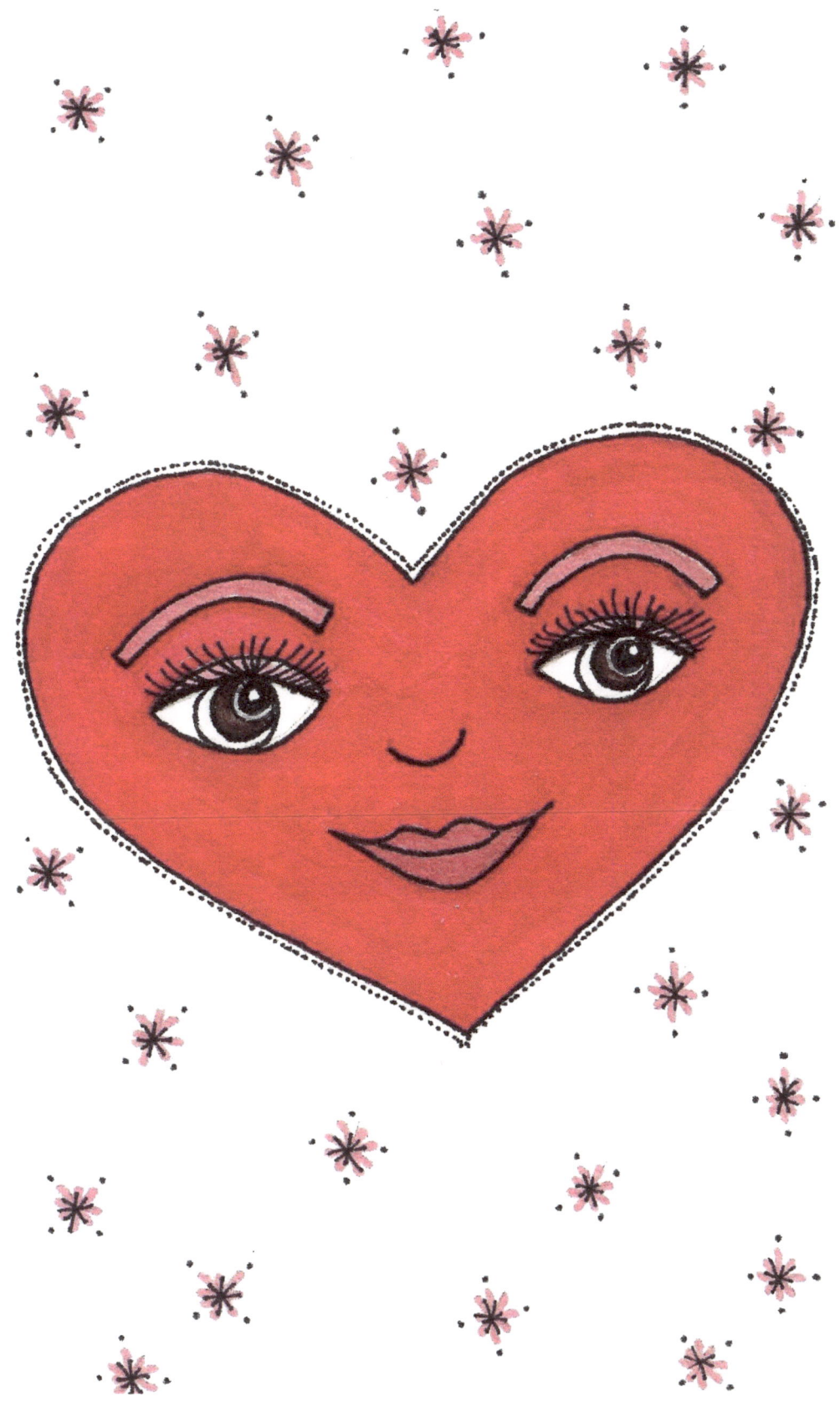

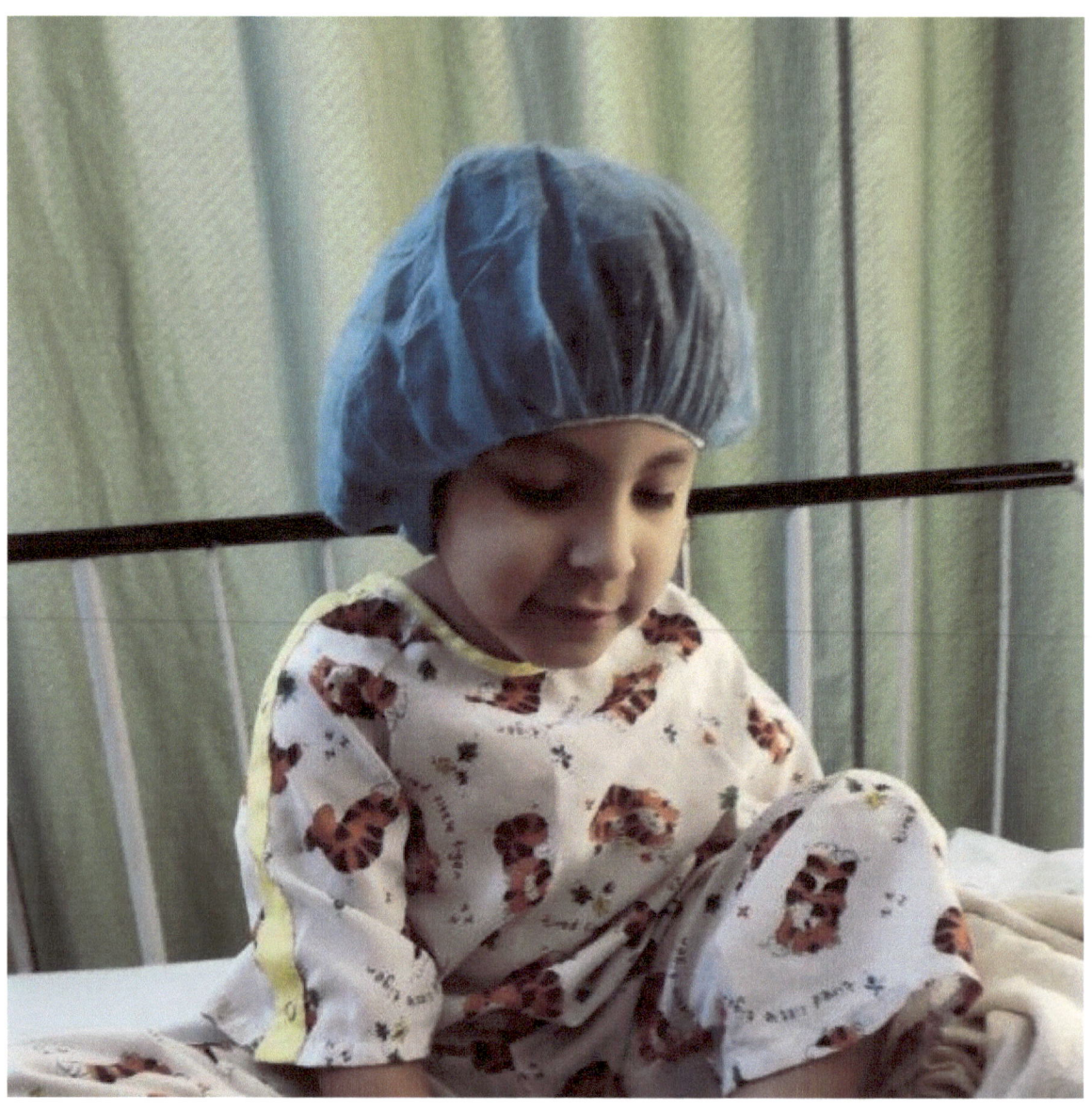

Audrey was born in 2013 with a ventricular septal defect (VSD) which is a small hole in heart. Most children have this corrected right after birth with no memory of the surgery other than the scar on their chest. It wasn't until Audrey was four years old, that her VSD started to affect her aortic valve requiring surgery to repair it. How do you explain open heart surgery to a four-year-old? This was during her princess glitter phase, so I sat her down and explained that her glitter was leaking from her heart so the doctors need to save her glitter because that's what makes her sparkle! And that is how The Glitter Heart story was born. Till this day, if someone asks about her scar, she says, "oh, that's from when they saved my glitter!"

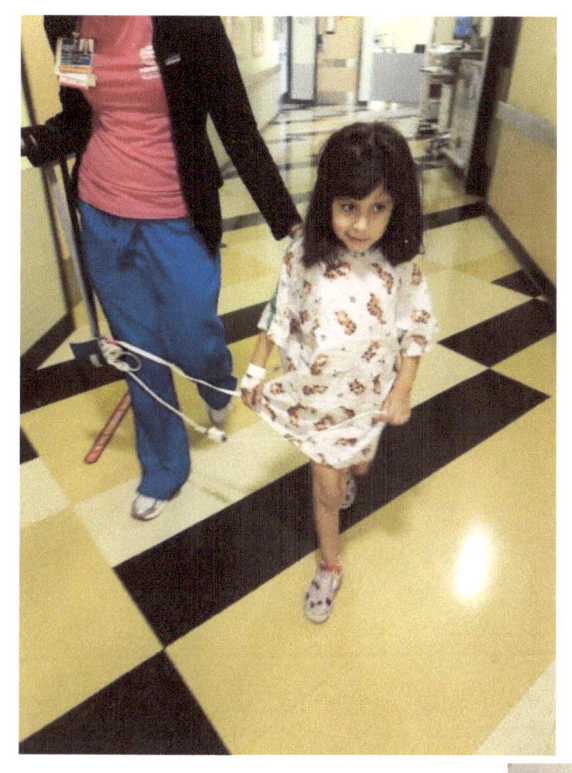

Remember to be Brave and Sparkle on!

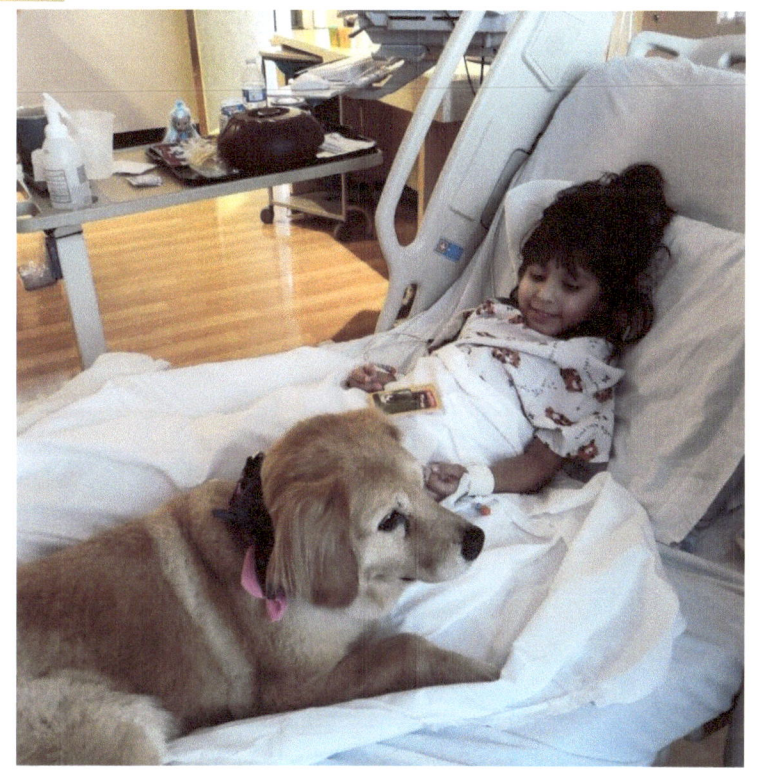

www.ingramcontent.com/pod-product-compliance
Lightning Source LLC
Chambersburg PA
CBHW051836210526
45473CB00005B/1906